The Ult
Ketogenic Desserts Cookbook

Delicious Low-Carbs, High Protein Desserts Recipes

By

Elisa Hayes

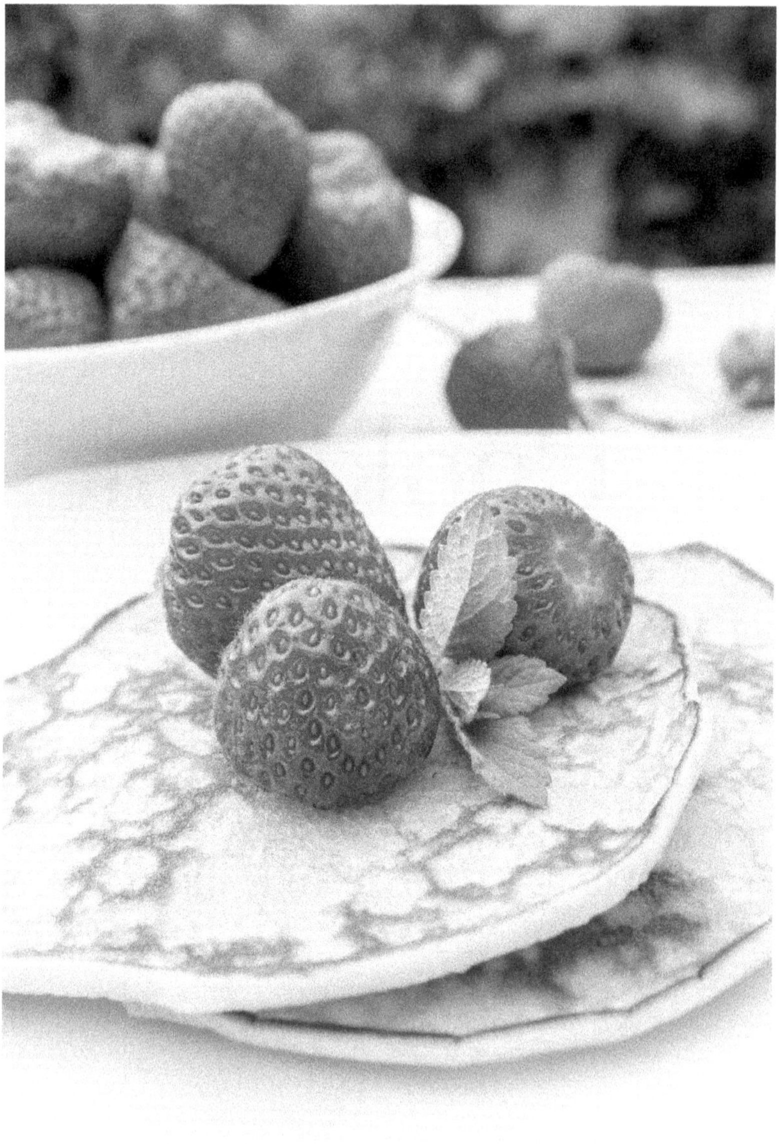

Table of Contents

The information in the following pages is broadly considered a truthful and accurate account of facts and as such, any inattention, use, or misuse of the information in question by the reader will render any resulting actions solely under their purview. There are no scenarios in which the publisher or the original author of this work can be in any fashion deemed liable for any hardship or damages that may befall them after undertaking information described herein.

Additionally, the information in the following pages is intended only for informational purposes and should thus be thought of as universal. As befitting its nature, it is presented without assurance regarding its prolonged validity or interim quality. Trademarks that are mentioned are done without written consent and can in no way be considered an endorsement from the trademark holder.

Introduction

The path to a perfect body and good physical health was very thorny for me. The only one wish which I was making for my birthdays for many years was to be a slim and beautiful girl. Alas, everything can't be as in fairy tales and the miracle didn't happen; my mirror was still showing the same fat, pimple girl. In childhood, the problem of being overweight didn't bother me much; I can say that I didn't care about it at all, I didn't know that weight would be momentous for me. I was an ordinary smiling child, playing with my peers, going to school, and traveling with my parents. That time my chubby cheeks seemed very sweet to everyone. But that was then. At 11-year-old, I went to middle school. New people, new teachers, I had no friends at all. Mentally I was broken. I counted the minutes until the end of the last lesson, to quickly sit in my mom's car and leave school. I started to eat a lot. Now I see that in this way I am stressed, but then the food served as my antidepressant. Dozens of hamburgers, fried potatoes, coke – they were "my best friends". In addition to everything, I started to have horrible skin problems, it seemed to me that there was no place on my face wherever they hadn't appeared yet. Time passed and I no longer loved my reflection in the mirror even in 1%. I couldn't wear the clothes that I liked. I usually wore oversized shorts and t-shirts. I couldn't afford to wear a short dress and high heels. At 15-year-old I weighed more than 270lbs. I remember what I felt in those days, as it is happening now. I felt anger, irritation, hatred, and self-loathing. That prom party was the most terrible day of my life. Thank God it's over!

In those years, the keto diet was not very popular, fasting and drinking diets (which, as you already know, did not help me much) were more popular. Perhaps I wouldn't do anything, but my health problems were becoming more serious. It seemed that my body was simply screaming: please help me!

I remember the day that changed my life on a dime. I came to the clinic with pain in my stomach. But this time, I not only received painkillers but also found a mentor and friend. This was my physician. She had examined me and recommended that I go on a diet. I didn't want to do something and was categorically against it. However, my mind changed when she said: love your body, care about it, and it will thank you. What was my surprise when the diet turned out to be very simple to follow. Is it so easy to love myself? As you could understand I am talking about my favorite keto diet. Every day I was eating a maximum of proteins and a minimum of carbohydrates. That meant to consume meat, poultry, and fish and make restrictions for vegetables, fruits, and sweets. After 2 weeks, I lost 83lbs, and further results were getting better and better. All this time I was under the supervision of a doctor and this yielded results. A year later, I completely changed all the clothes in my wardrobe and oh my God I was able to wear a short dress and skirts! Now I can say that I am the happiest person. It happened because I fell in love with myself and started treating my body as a diamond. My life was filled with bright colors, I have a beloved husband, children, work, friends, I am healthy and like myself in the mirror. I am telling this story to prove that the right diet can solve almost all problems with body and health. It is a fact that our body is capable of dealing with dramatic changes, it is only worth loving it. Never rest on your laurels, never give up and forbid people to say that you cannot do something. You are already a great fellow that you bought this cookbook and decided to take a step ahead in the direction to your dream. Let this book become your ray of hope, a lifesaver on the way to your wonderful transformation. If you believe in yourself and love your body, believe me, the result won't be long in coming. You will see in the mirror a completely new version of yourself, updated physically and mentally! Just trust the keto diet and your inner voice. Set a goal today and start the way of achieving it right now. Don't try to do it all in one time; let it be a small step day by day. Exactly now, this is the right time to start creating a new version of you. If this diet was able to change my life, I'm sure it will help you too!

Chocolate Pie

Prep time: 10 minutes

Cook time: 30 minutes

Servings: 8

Ingredients:

- 3 tablespoons butter, softened
- ½ cup heavy cream
- 1 teaspoon baking powder
- 1 cup coconut flour
- 1 oz dark chocolate, chopped

Method:

1. Mix butter with baking powder, coconut flour, and heavy cream.
2. Then transfer the mixture in the non-stick baking pan. Flatten the surface of the pie with the help of the spatula and top with chopped chocolate.
3. Bake the pie at 360F for 30 minutes.

Nutritional info per serve: Calories 91, Fat 8.4, Fiber 0.8, Carbs 3.6, Protein 0.7

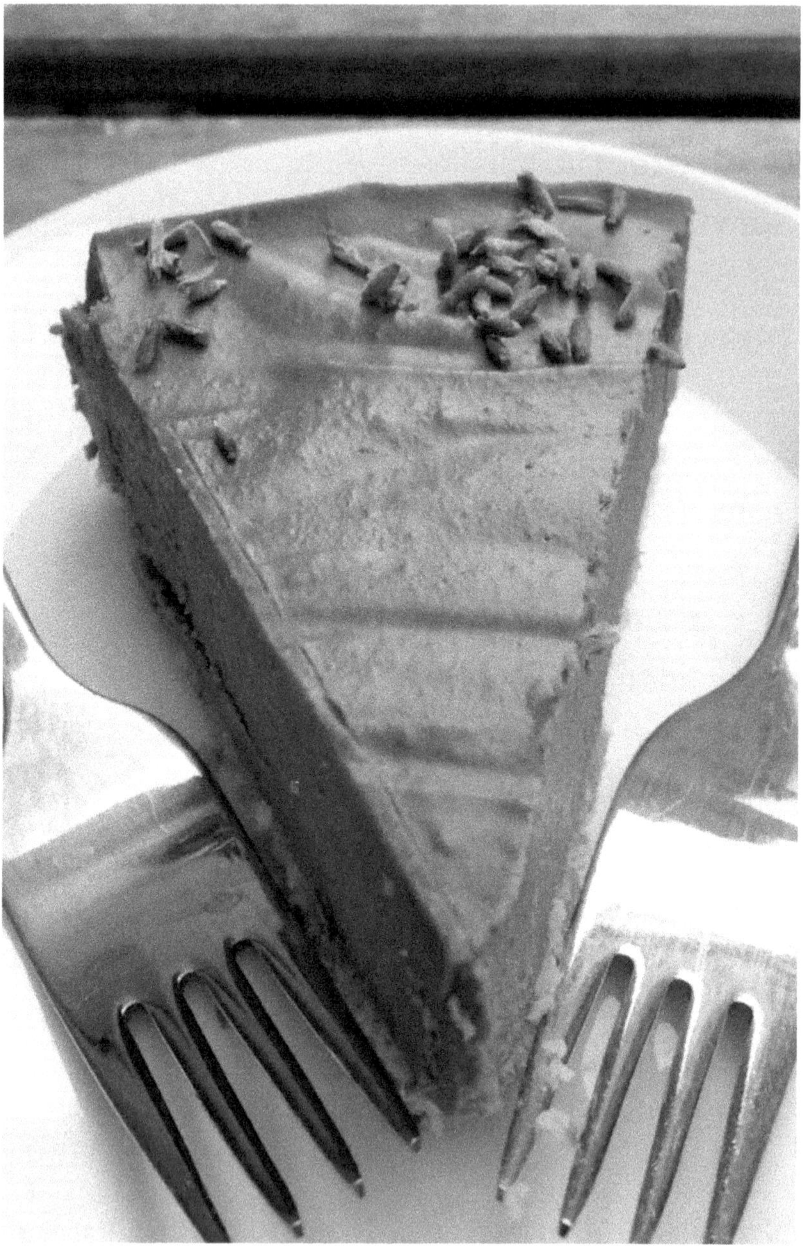

Coconut Panna Cotta

Prep time: 40 minutes

Cook time: 10 minutes

Servings:2

Ingredients:

- 1 cup coconut cream
- 1 teaspoon vanilla extract
- 2 teaspoons Erythritol
- 2 teaspoon coconut shred
- 1 tablespoon gelatin powder

Method:

1. Mix coconut cream with gelatin powder, vanilla extract, and Erythritol and preheat for 4 minutes.
2. Whisk the mixture until gelatin is dissolved and pour it in the serving cups.
3. Top every cup with coconut shred and refrigerate for 40 minutes.

Nutritional info per serve: Calories 310, Fat 30.3, Fiber 3, Carbs 7.6, Protein 5.8

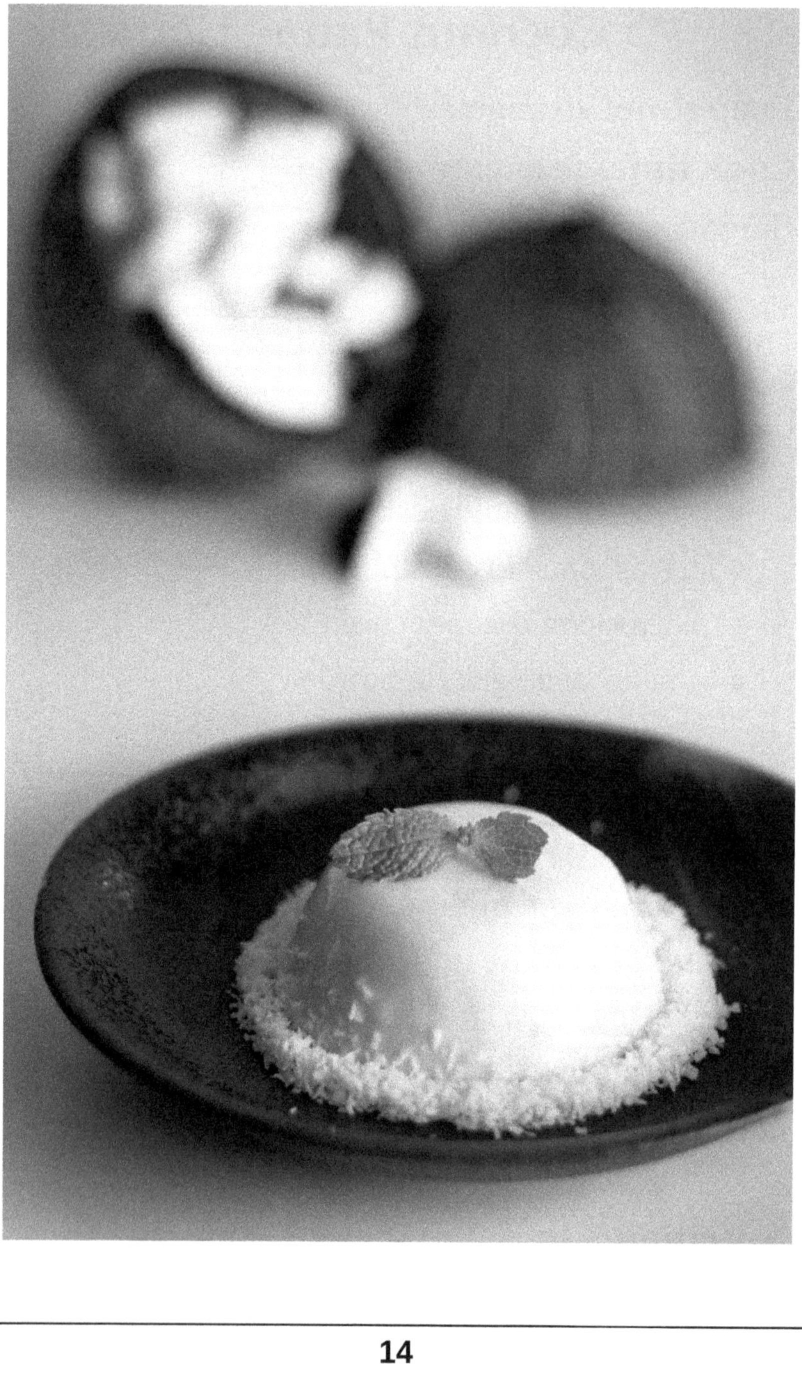

No-Baked Cheesecake

Prep time: 45 minutes

Cook time: 1 minute

Servings: 8

Ingredients:

- 1 cup cream cheese
- 3 tablespoons Erythritol
- 1 tablespoon gelatin
- 5 tablespoons water

Method:

1. Mix gelatin with water and leave for 10 minutes. Then microwave the mixture for 1 minute or until it is liquid.
2. After this, mix cream cheese with liquid gelatin and Erythritol.
3. Pour the cheesecake mixture in the cheesecake mold and refrigerate for 30-40 minutes or until the cheesecake is solid.

Nutritional info per serve: Calories 104, Fat 10.1, Fiber 0, Carbs 0.8, Protein 2.9

Coconut Cookies

Prep time: 15 minutes

Cook time: 13 minutes

Servings:6

Ingredients:

- ½ cup coconut flour
- 2 teaspoons coconut oil
- ¾ teaspoon coconut shred
- 1 teaspoon Erythritol
- 3 tablespoons coconut milk

Method:

1. In the mixing bowl, mix coconut flour with coconut oil, coconut shred, and Erythritol.
2. Add coconut milk and knead the dough.
3. Then make 6 balls from the dough and press them gently in the shape of the cookies.
4. Bake the cookies at 360F for 13 minutes.

Nutritional info per serve: Calories 37, Fat 3.7, Fiber 0.6, Carbs 1.2, Protein 0.3

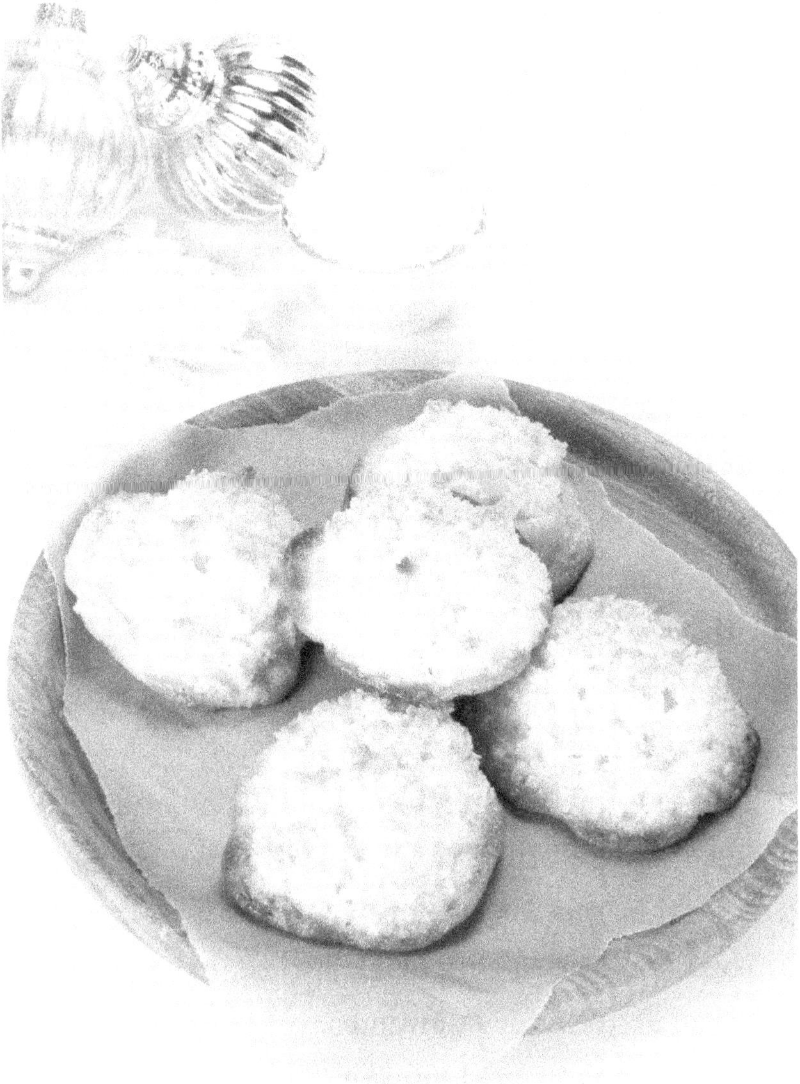

Blackberries Bars

Prep time: 10 minutes

Cook time: 15 minutes

Servings: 12

Ingredients:

- ½ cup butter
- 2 oz blackberries, chopped
- 2 tablespoons Erythritol
- 2 tablespoons coconut flour
- ½ cup coconut, shredded

Method:

1. Mix butter with coconut flour and coconut shred and knead the dough.
2. Then put the mixture in the baking pan and flatten in the shape of the pie crust.
3. After this, mix blackberries with Erythritol.
4. Top the pie crust with blackberries mixture and bake in the oven at 360F for 15 minutes.
5. Cut the cooked meal into bars.

Nutritional info per serve: Calories 87, Fat 9, Fiber 1.1, Carbs 1.7, Protein 0.5

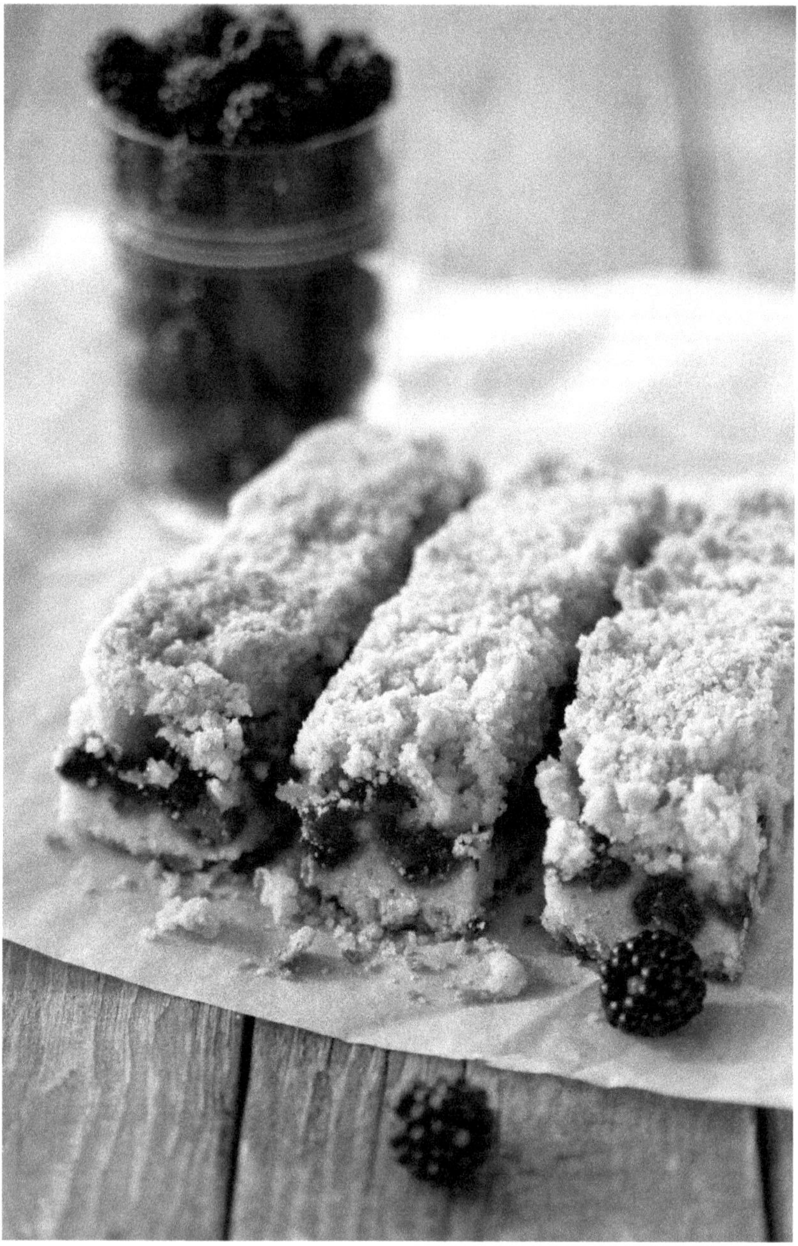

Cheesecake Bars

Prep time: 25 minutes

Cook time: 10 minutes

Servings:8

Ingredients:

- 1 cup cream cheese
- 3 egg, beaten
- ¼ cup of coconut milk
- 3 tablespoons Erythritol
- 1 teaspoon vanilla extract
- ¼ cup coconut flour
- 1 tablespoon butter
- 1 tablespoon flax meal

Method:

1. In the mixing bowl, mix eggs with coconut milk, Erythritol, vanilla extract, coconut flour, butter, and flax meal.
2. Put the mixture in the baking pan and flatten in the shape of the pie crust.
3. Then bake it at 360F for 10 minutes.

4. Chill the cooked pie crust well and spread it with cream cheese.
5. Cut the meal into bars.

Nutritional info per serve: Calories 162, Fat 15.4, Fiber 0.6, Carbs 1.9, Protein 4.7

Cocoa Muffins

Prep time: 30 minutes

Cook time: 12 minutes

Servings: 6

Ingredients:

- 6 teaspoons butter
- 1 egg, beaten
- 2 tablespoons Erythritol
- 2 teaspoons cocoa powder
- 1 cup coconut flour

Method:

1. Put all ingredients in the mixing bowl and whisk until you get a smooth batter.
2. After this, pour the batter in the muffin molds (fill ½ part of every mold) and bake at 365F for 12 minutes.
3. Cool the cooked muffins and remove them from the molds.

Nutritional info per serve: Calories 126, Fat 6.6, Fiber 8.2, Carbs 13.7, Protein 3.7

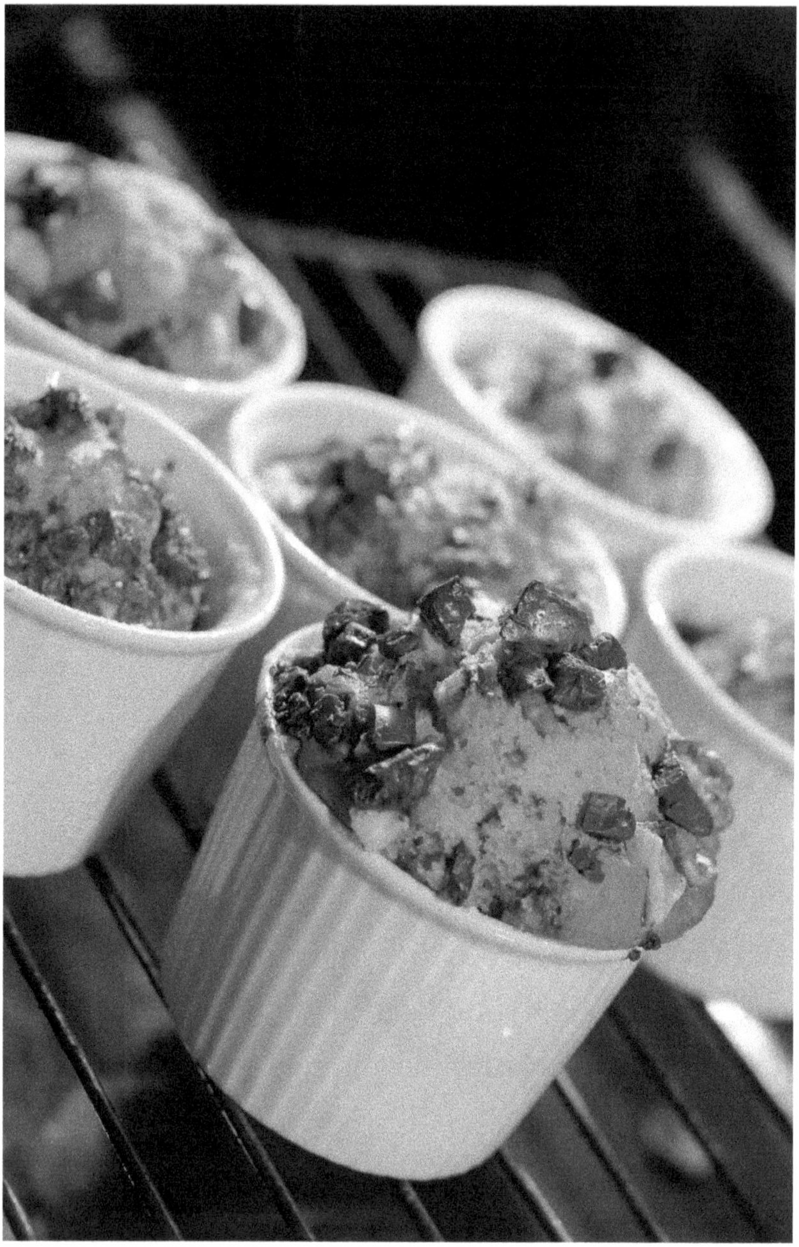

Coconut Pudding

Prep time: 20 minutes

Cook time: 10 minutes

Servings:2

Ingredients:

- ½ cup coconut cream
- 2 eggs, beaten
- 1 teaspoon coconut flour
- 2 tablespoons Erythritol
- 1 teaspoon vanilla extract

Method:

1. Mix all ingredients in the saucepan and stir until smooth.
2. Bring the liquid to boil and remove from the heat.
3. Transfer it in the serving cups and refrigerate for 15-20 minutes.

Nutritional info per serve: Calories 212, Fat 18.8, Fiber 1.7, Carbs 4.6, Protein 7.1

Cream Cheese Mousse

Prep time: 10 minutes

Cook time: 0 minutes

Servings: 2

Ingredients:

- ½ cup coconut cream
- 3 tablespoons cream cheese
- 1 tablespoon Erythritol
- 1 tablespoon coconut shred

Method:

1. Mix coconut cream with coconut shred, Erythritol, and cream cheese.
2. Whisk the mixture until it is soft and fluffy.
3. Transfer the mousse in the serving cups.

Nutritional info per serve: Calories 238, Fat 23.8, Fiber 2.3, Carbs 5.7, Protein 3

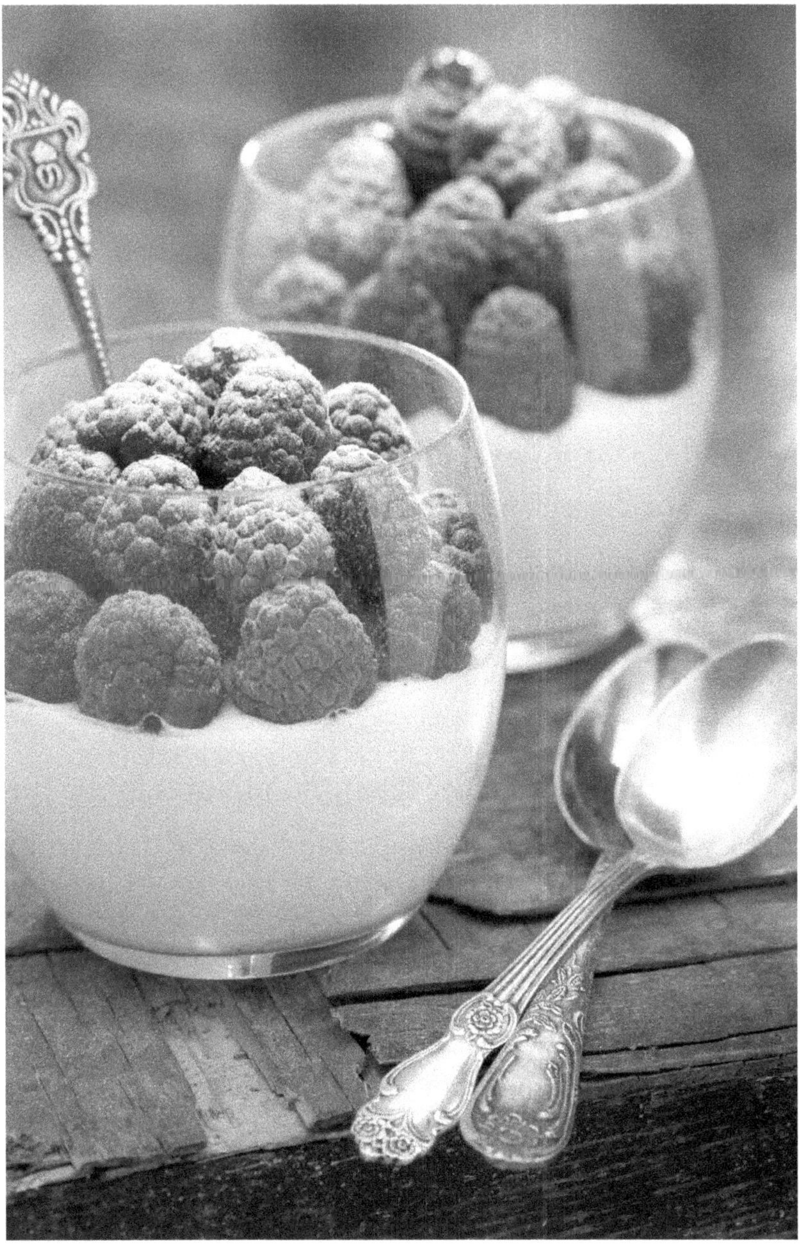

Chocolate Bacon Strips

Prep time: 30 minutes

Cook time: 5 minutes

Servings:6

Ingredients:

- 6 bacon sliced, cooked
- 2 oz dark chocolate
- 1 tablespoon coconut oil
- ¼ teaspoon dried mint

Method:

1. Freeze the bacon slices for 15-20 minutes in the freezer.
2. Meanwhile, melt chocolate and mix it with coconut oil and dried mint.
3. Then dip every bacon slice in the chocolate mixture and refrigerate for 10-15 minutes.

Nutritional info per serve: Calories 173, Fat 13, Fiber 0.3, Carbs 5.9, Protein 7.8

Cocoa Fudge

Prep time: 10 minutes

Cook time: 30 minutes

Servings: 4

Ingredients:

- 4 tablespoons coconut oil
- ¼ cup of coconut milk
- ½ teaspoon vanilla extract
- 2 teaspoons Erythritol
- 3 tablespoons cocoa powder

Method:

1. Melt the coconut oil and mix it with cocoa powder, Erythritol, vanilla extract, and coconut milk. Stir the mixture until homogenous.
2. Then line the baking mold with baking paper.
3. Pour the fudge mixture inside, flatten it and refrigerate for 30 minutes.
4. Cut the fudge into bars.

Nutritional info per serve: Calories 162, Fat 17.7, Fiber 1.5, Carbs 3.1, Protein 1.1

Sweet Mousse

Prep time: 10 minutes

Cook time: 10 minutes

Servings: 5

Ingredients:

- 1 cup heavy cream
- 1 tablespoon Erythritol
- 5 teaspoons cream cheese
- 1 tablespoon coconut flour

Method:

1. Bring the heavy cream to boil and add coconut flour and Erythritol.
2. Simmer the cream mixture for 30 seconds.
3. Then add cream cheese and whisk the mousse until it is smooth.
4. Transfer it in the serving cups.

Nutritional info per serve: Calories 100, Fat 10.2, Fiber 0.5, Carbs 4.6, Protein 0.9

Lemon Pie

Prep time: 15 minutes

Cook time: 25 minutes

Servings:6

Ingredients:

- ½ lemon, chopped
- 1 cup almond flour
- ¼ cup of coconut oil
- ¼ cup of coconut milk
- 1 teaspoon baking powder
- 3 tablespoons Erythritol

Method:

1. Mix almond flour with coconut oil, coconut milk, baking powder, and Erythritol.
2. Transfer the mixture in the non-stick baking pan and top with chopped lemon.
3. Bake the pie at 360F for 25 minutes.
4. Then cool the pie well and cut into servings.

Nutritional info per serve: Calories 130, Fat 13.8, Fiber 0.9, Carbs 9.9, Protein 1.3

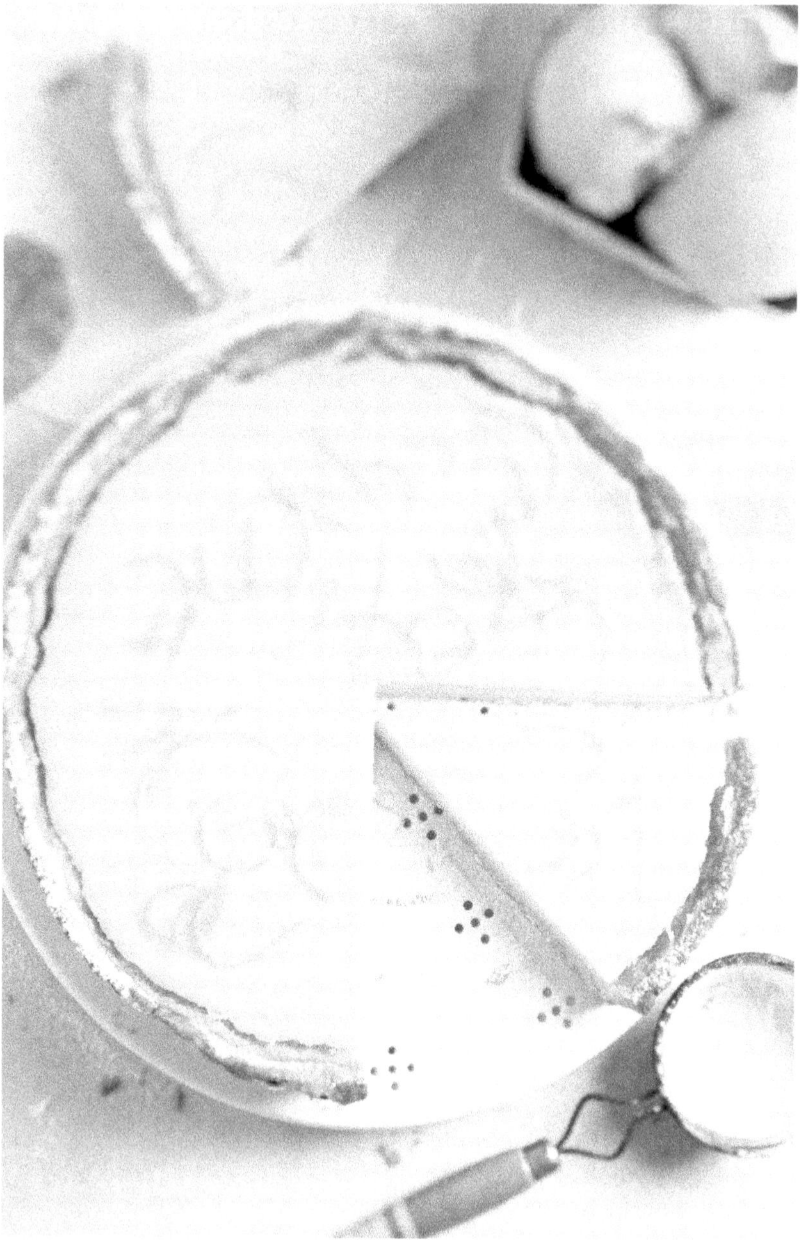

2-Ingredients Ice Cream

Prep time: 10 minutes

Cook time: 0 minutes

Servings: 2

Ingredients:

- 2 raspberries, frozen
- 2 blackberries, frozen

Method:

1. Put the raspberries and blackberries in the food processor and blend until smooth.
2. Transfer the mixture in the serving glasses.

Nutritional info per serve: Calories 10, Fat 0.1, Fiber 1.3, Carbs 2.4, Protein 0.2

Berry Muffins

Prep time: 10 minutes

Cook time: 14 minutes

Servings:8

Ingredients:

- 1/3 cup coconut oil
- 1 teaspoon vanilla extract
- 2 tablespoons Erythritol
- 1 cup coconut flour
- 1 oz raspberries
- 1 egg, beaten
- 1 teaspoon baking powder

Method:

1. Put all ingredients except raspberries in the mixing bowl and mix until smooth.
2. Then add raspberries and carefully mix the muffin batter with the help of the spoon.
3. Transfer the mixture in the muffin molds (fill ½ part of every mold) and bake at 365F for 14 minutes.

Nutritional info per serve: Calories 150, Fat 11.2, Fiber 6.2, Carbs 14.6, Protein 2.7

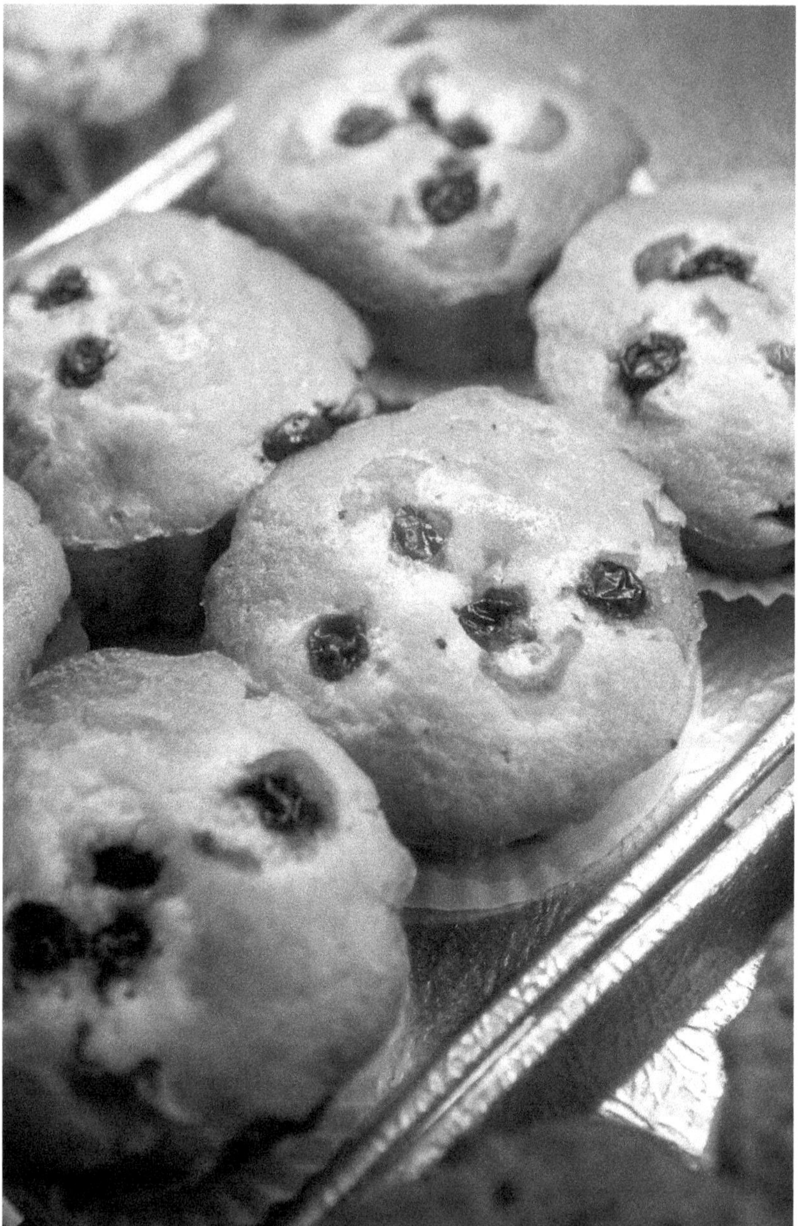

Cocoa Squares

Prep time: 10 minutes

Cook time: 21 minutes

Servings: 9

Ingredients:

- 4 tablespoons butter, softened
- ½ teaspoon baking powder
- 4 tablespoons Erythritol
- 1 teaspoon vanilla extract
- 4 ounces cream cheese
- 6 eggs, beaten
- 3 tablespoons cocoa powder

Method:

1. Mix butter with baking powder, Erythritol, vanilla extract, cream cheese, eggs, and cocoa powder.
2. When the mixture is homogeneous, transfer it in the baking pan and bake for 21 minutes at 360F.

Nutritional info per serve: Calories 137, Fat 12.7, Fiber 0.6, Carbs 8.4, Protein 5

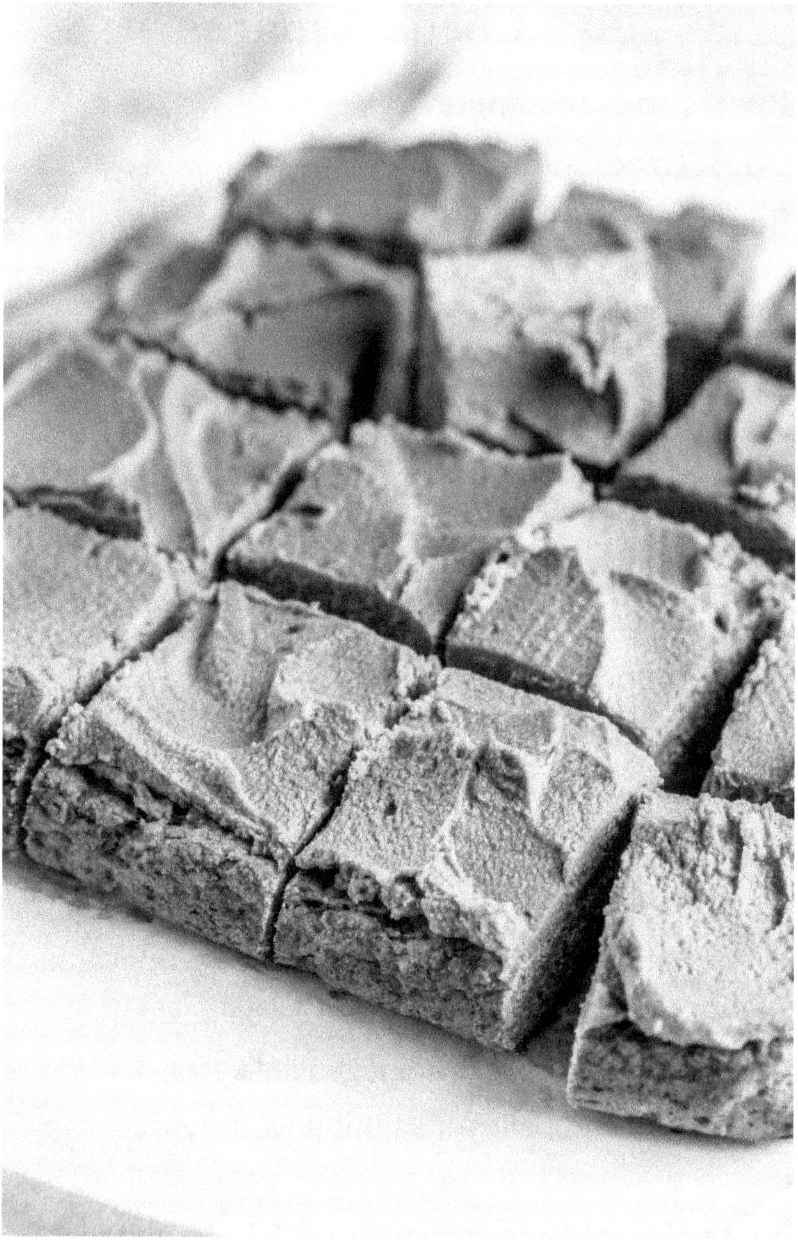

Avocado Pie

Prep time: 10 minutes

Cook time: 30 minutes

Servings:6

Ingredients:

- 1 avocado, pitted, peeled, sliced
- 1 cup heavy cream
- 1 ½ cup coconut flour
- 1 teaspoon baking powder
- 3 tablespoons Erythritol
- 1 tablespoon butter

Method:

1. Mix coconut flour with heavy cream, baking powder, Erythritol, and butter.
2. Make the smooth mixture and pour it in the non-stick baking pan.
3. Top the batter with avocado and bake at 360F for 30 minutes.

Nutritional info per serve: Calories 275, Fat 18.9, Fiber 14.3, Carbs 23.8, Protein 5.1

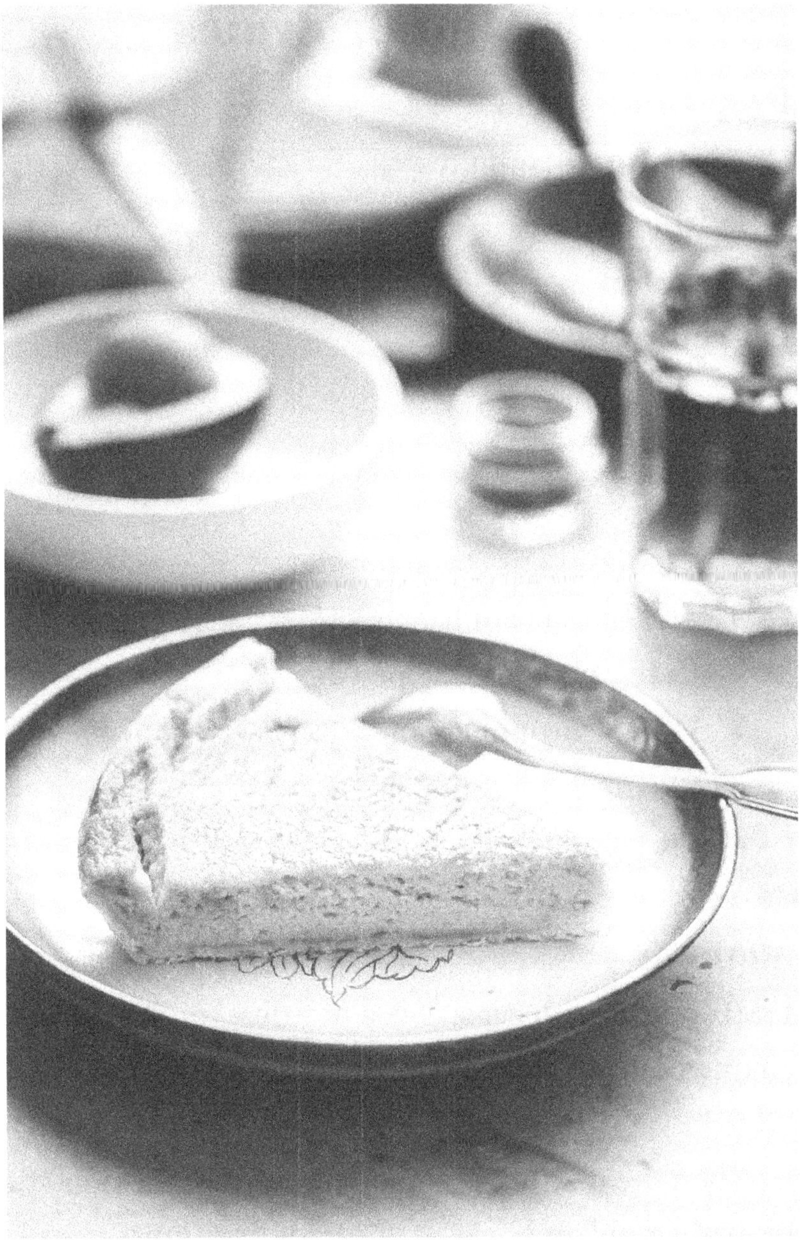

Mint Brownies

Prep time: 10 minutes

Cook time: 35 minutes

Servings: 12

Ingredients:

- 1 cup butter
- 6 eggs, beaten
- 3 tablespoons cocoa powder
- 1 teaspoon vanilla extract
- ½ teaspoon baking powder
- ½ cup coconut cream
- ½ cup coconut flour
- 1 teaspoon dried mint

Method:

1. Mix butter with eggs, cocoa powder, vanilla extract, baking powder, coconut cream, coconut flour, and dried mint.
2. When the mixture is smooth, pour it in the non-sticky brownie mold and bake at 360F for 35 minutes.
3. Cut the brownie into bars when they are cooked.

Nutritional info per serve: Calories 214, Fat 20.6, Fiber 2.6, Carbs 5, Protein 4.1

Almond Bars

Prep time: 15 minutes

Cook time: 12 minutes

Servings:4

Ingredients:

- ½ cup almond flour
- 2 oz almonds, chopped
- 3 tablespoons butter
- 1 tablespoon Erythritol
- 1 teaspoon vanilla extract
- ½ teaspoon baking powder

Method:

1. Mix almond flour with butter, Erythritol, vanilla extract, and baking powder.
2. Then add almond and knead the dough.
3. Put the dough in the lined with the baking paper tray and cut into bars.
4. Bake the dessert for 12 minutes at 360F.

Nutritional info per serve: Calories 643, Fat 61.8, Fiber 7.9, Carbs 14.9, Protein 12.2

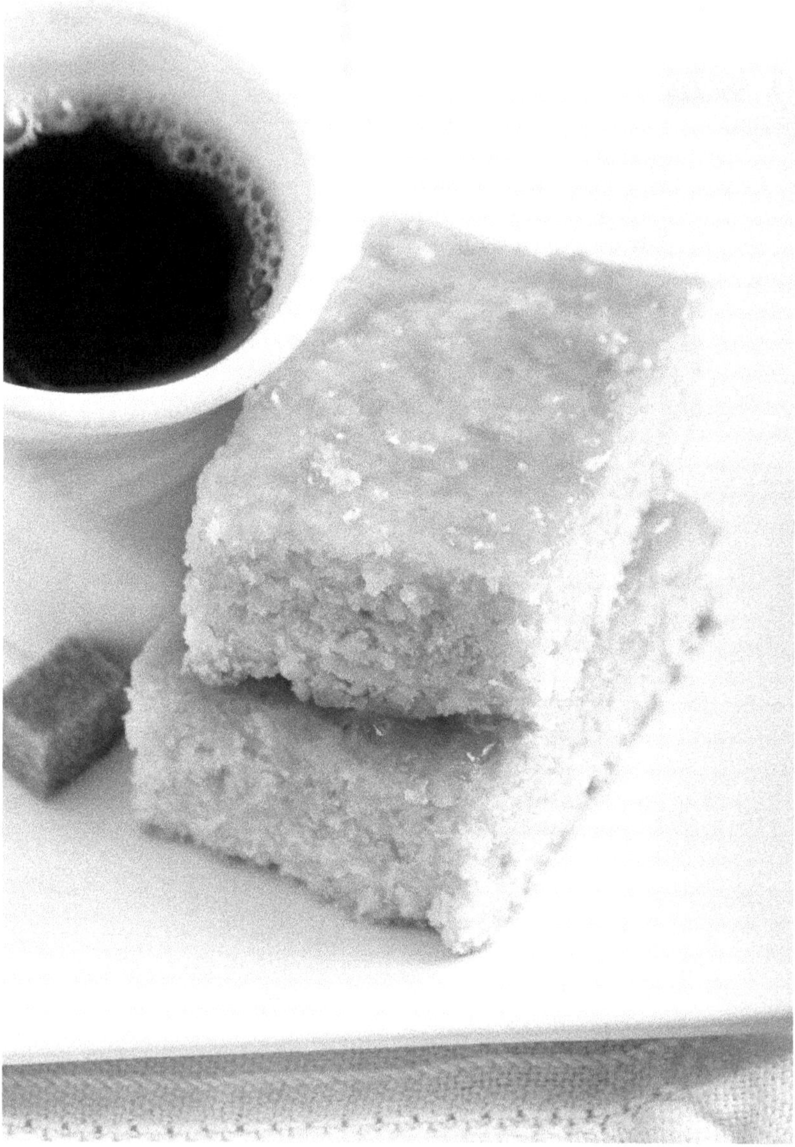

Coconut Chia Pudding

Cook time: 30 minutes

Servings: 2

Ingredients:

- 1 cup of coconut milk
- 1 tablespoon coconut shred
- 3 tablespoons chia seeds

Method:

1. Mix coconut milk with coconut shred and chia seeds.
2. Transfer the mixture in the servings glasses and leave for 25 minutes to rest.

Nutritional info per serve: Calories 404, Fat 37.6, Fiber 10.4, Carbs 16.6, Protein 6.3

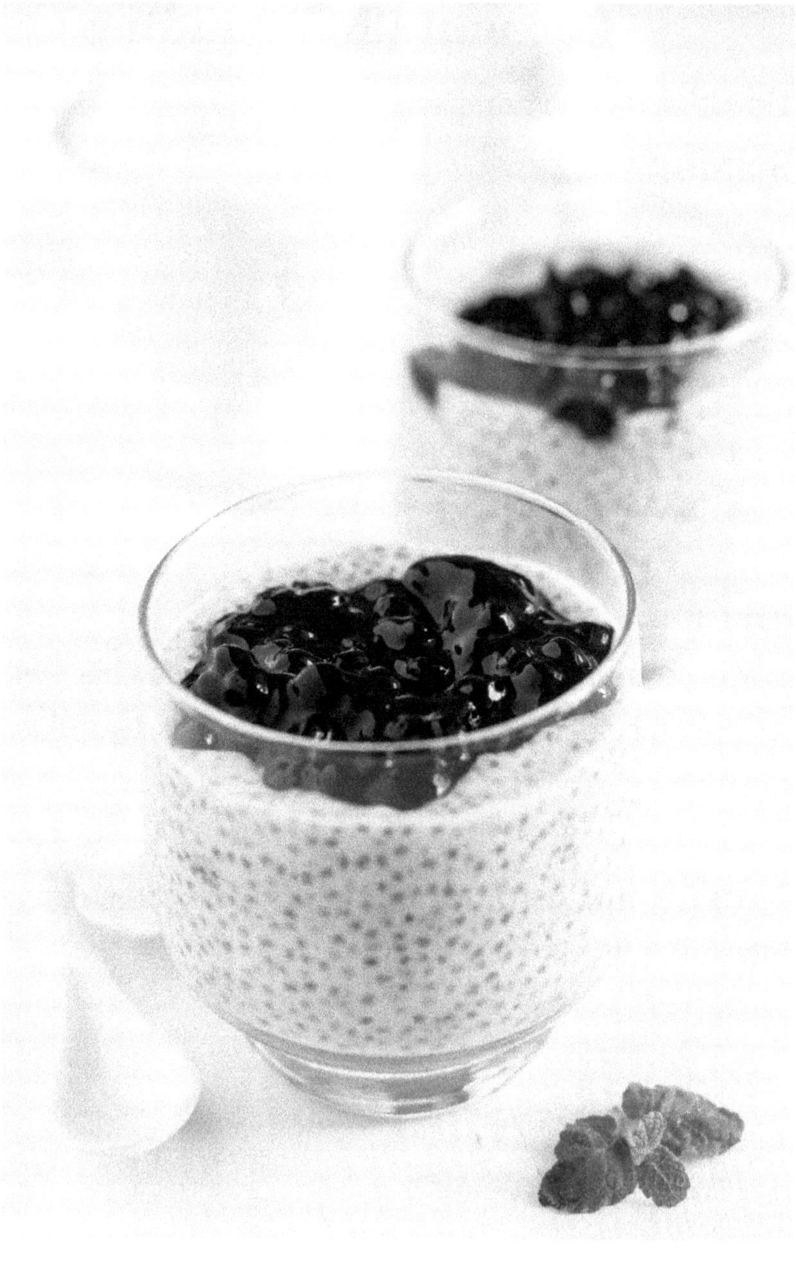

Matcha Muffins

Prep time: 10 minutes

Cook time: 14 minutes

Servings:5

Ingredients:

- 1 teaspoon matcha tea
- 1 teaspoon baking powder
- 1 cup of coconut milk
- 1 cup coconut flour
- 1 teaspoon vanilla extract
- 1 tablespoon butter, melted

Method:

1. In the mixing bowl, mix matcha tea with baking powder, coconut milk, coconut flour, vanilla extract, and butter.
2. Stir the mixture until you get a smooth batter and pour it in the muffin molds.
3. Bake the muffins at 360F for 14 minutes.

Nutritional info per serve: Calories 231, Fat 16.1, Fiber 10.7, Carbs 19.4, Protein 4.3

Coconut Parfaits

Prep time: 10 minutes

Cook time: 0 minutes

Servings: 6

Ingredients:

- 2 cups of coconut milk
- 1 teaspoon vanilla extract
- 2 tablespoons Erythritol
- 4 strawberries, chopped
- 4 pecans, chopped

Method:

1. Mix coconut milk with vanilla extract and Erythritol.
2. Then put strawberries in every serving glass.
3. Top them with coconut milk and pecans.

Nutritional info per serve: Calories 254, Fat 25.8, Fiber 2.9, Carbs 11.5, Protein 2.9

Vanilla Shake

Prep time: 5 minutes

Cook time: 3 minutes

Servings:4

Ingredients:

- 2 cups of coconut milk
- 1 avocado, pitted, peeled, chopped
- 1 teaspoon vanilla extract
- 1 tablespoon Erythritol

Method:

1. Put all ingredients in the food processor and blend for 3 minutes.
2. Pour the vanilla shake in the glasses.

Nutritional info per serve: Calories 382, Fat 38.4, Fiber 6, Carbs 14.9, Protein 3.7

Lemon Pudding

Prep time: 10 minutes

Cook time: 10 minutes

Servings:4

Ingredients:

- 2 cups of coconut milk
- 1 teaspoon lemon zest
- 1 teaspoon vanilla extract
- 3 egg yolks
- 1 tablespoon Erythritol

Method:

1. Mix coconut milk with egg yolks and vanilla extract.
2. Bring the liquid to boil. Stir it constantly.
3. Then add Erythritol and lemon zest.
4. Whisk the pudding and transfer it in the serving glasses. Chill the pudding to the room temperature.

Nutritional info per serve: Calories 320, Fat 32, Fiber 2.7, Carbs 11.1, Protein 4.8

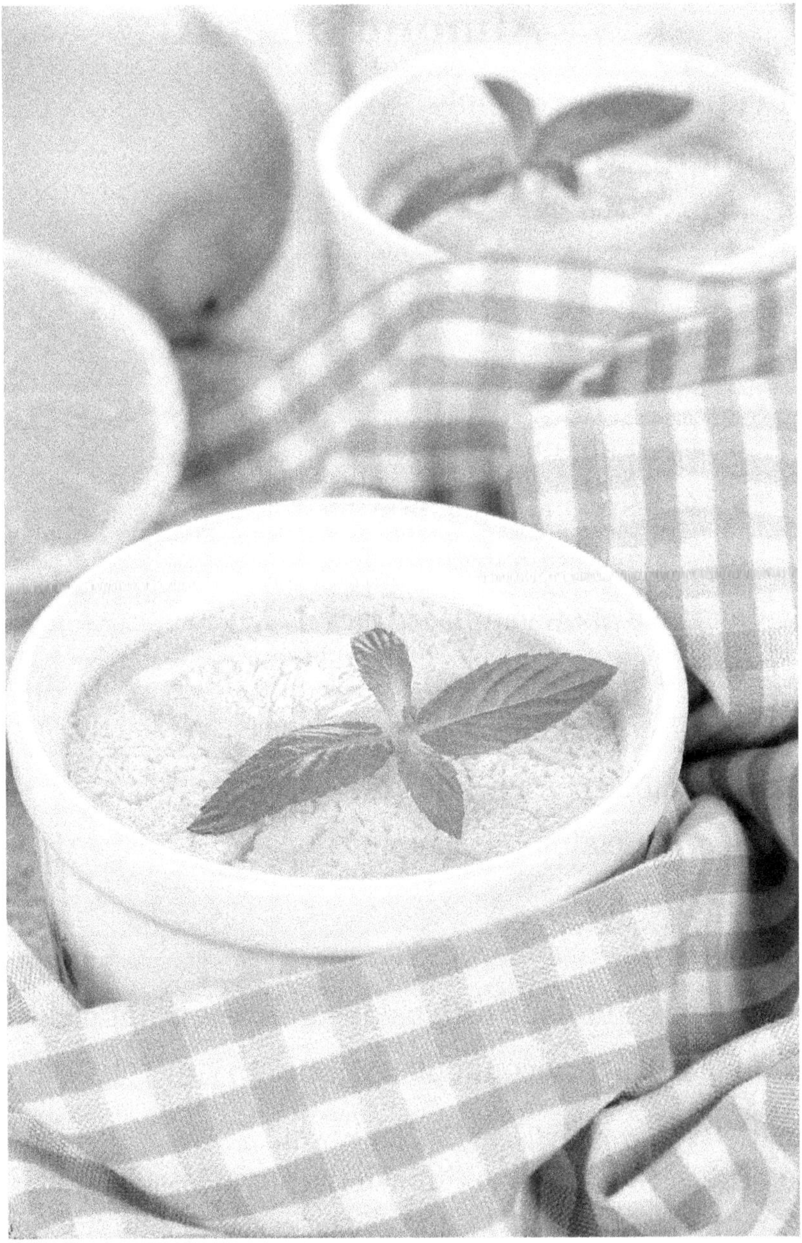

Almond Biscotti

Prep time: 10 minutes

Cook time: 30 minutes

Servings:7

Ingredients:

- 1 cup almond flour
- 1 teaspoon baking powder
- 1/3 teaspoon ground clove
- 1 teaspoon vanilla extract
- 2 tablespoons coconut oil
- 1 egg, beaten
- 1 tablespoon Erythritol
- ¼ cup almonds, chopped

Method:

1. Mix almond flour with baking powder, ground clove, vanilla extract, coconut oil, egg, and Erythritol. Add almonds.
2. Knead the dough and make the shape of loaf from it.
3. Then put it in the preheated to 365F oven and bake for 20 minutes.

4. Then slice the cooked loaf into pieces and return to the oven. Put the sliced loaf in one layer.
5. Cook the dessert at 360F for 10 minutes more.
6. Chill the cooked biscotti well.

Nutritional info per serve: Calories 156, Fat 14.2, Fiber 2.2, Carbs 6.8, Protein 5

Peppermint Cream

Prep time: 20 minutes

Cook time: 0 minutes

Servings: 3

Ingredients:

- ½ cup butter softened
- 1 tablespoon Erythritol
- 1 tablespoon cocoa powder
- 1 avocado, pitted, peeled, chopped
- 2 tablespoons ricotta cheese

Method:

1. Mix butter with cocoa powder.
2. Then add Erythritol, avocado, and ricotta cheese.
3. Blend the mixture until you get smooth and soft cream.

Nutritional info per serve: Calories 426, Fat 44.8, Fiber 5, Carbs 12.3, Protein 3.1

Zucchini Pudding

Prep time: 15 minutes

Cook time: 10 minutes

Servings:6

Ingredients:

- 1 zucchini, grated
- 2 eggs, whisked
- ½ teaspoon baking powder
- ½ cup coconut cream
- 1 cup coconut flour
- 2 tablespoons Erythritol
- ½ teaspoon vanilla extract
- ¾ teaspoon ground cardamom

Method:

1. Put all ingredients in the food processor and blend until smooth.
2. Then transfer the mixture in the saucepan and simmer for 5 minutes.
3. Cool the cooked pudding and transfer it in the serving glasses.

Nutritional info per serve: Calories 154, Fat 8.3, Fiber 8.9, Carbs 21.1, Protein 5.4

Egg Pudding

Prep time: 10 minutes

Cook time: 10 minutes

Servings: 6

Ingredients:

- 1 ⅔ cups of coconut milk
- 5 eggs, beaten
- 5 tablespoons Erythritol
- 1 teaspoon vanilla extract

Method:

1. Mix eggs with coconut milk, Erythritol, and vanilla extract.
2. Pour the liquid in the saucepan and simmer it for 10 minutes on low heat.
3. Chill the pudding and put it in the serving bowls.

Nutritional info per serve: Calories 208, Fat 19.5, Fiber 1.5, Carbs 6.6, Protein 6.1

Basil Cookies

Prep time: 15 minutes

Cook time: 15 minutes

Servings:6

Ingredients:

- 1 tablespoon dried basil
- 2 tablespoons Erythritol
- 1 tablespoon coconut oil, softened
- ½ cup coconut flour
- 3 tablespoons almond meal
- 2 tablespoons avocado oil

Method:

1. In the mixing bowl, mix dried basil, Erythritol, coconut oil, coconut flour, and almond meal.
2. Knead the dough and roll it up with the help of the rolling pin.
3. Then make the cookies with the help of the cutter.
4. Brush the baking tray with avocado oil.
5. Put the cookies inside and bake them for 15 minutes at 355F.

Nutritional info per serve: Calories 83, Fat 5.4, Fiber 4.6, Carbs 12.6, Protein 2

Clove Pudding

Prep time: 20 minutes

Cook time: 10 minutes

Servings: 2

Ingredients:

- 4 teaspoons gelatin
- ¼ teaspoon Erythritol
- 1 cup organic almond milk
- 1 teaspoon ground clove
- ¼ teaspoon ground cinnamon

Method:

1. Mix gelatin with almond milk and leave for 10 minutes.
2. Then stir the liquid, add ground clove, cinnamon, and Erythritol.
3. Bring the liquid to boil and remove from the heat.
4. Cool the pudding and pour it in the serving glasses.

Nutritional info per serve: Calories 327, Fat 28.8, Fiber 3.2, Carbs 8.2, Protein 14.8

Sweet Paprika Bars

Prep time: 20 minutes

Cook time: 15 minutes

Servings:4

Ingredients:

- 1 teaspoon pumpkin puree
- 1 egg, beaten
- ½ teaspoon vanilla extract
- ½ cup coconut flour
- ¼ teaspoon ground paprika
- 1 tablespoon ricotta cheese
- 1 tablespoon Erythritol

Method:

1. Mix pumpkin puree with egg, vanilla extract, coconut flour, ground paprika, ricotta cheese, and Erythritol.
2. Then transfer the mixture in the lined with the baking paper tray and flatten it if needed.
3. Bake the meal in the oven for 15 minutes at 360F.
4. Then remove the meal from the oven, cut into bars, and chill well.

Nutritional info per serve: Calories 83, Fat 2.9, Fiber 6.1, Carbs 14.3, Protein 3.9

Chia and Cocoa Biscuits

Prep time: 10 minutes

Cook time: 12 minutes

Servings: 8

Ingredients:

- 2 tablespoons chia seeds
- 2 cups coconut flour
- 1 egg, beaten
- ¼ cup butter, softened
- 2 tablespoons coconut, shredded
- 2 tablespoons Erythritol
- 1 tablespoon cocoa powder
- 1 teaspoon baking soda

Method:

1. Put all ingredients in the mixing bowl and knead the dough.
2. Then cut the dough into pieces and roll into balls.
3. Press the balls gently and put in the baking tray.
4. Bake the biscuits for 12 minutes at 365F.

Nutritional info per serve: Calories 219, Fat 12, Fiber 14.8, Carbs 27.3, Protein 6.1

Pecan Fudge

Prep time: 30 minutes

Cook time: 0 minutes

Servings:2

Ingredients:

- 1 oz dark chocolate (keto)
- ½ teaspoon of cocoa powder
- 2 tablespoons coconut oil
- 1 pecan, chopped

Method:

1. Melt the chocolate and mix it with coconut oil, cocoa powder, and pecan.
2. Whisk the mixture until smooth. Preheat it a little bit if needed.
3. Then pour the mixture in the silicone mold, flatten well and refrigerate for 20 minutes.
4. Cut the pecan fudge into pieces.

Nutritional info per serve: Calories 239, Fat 23.4, Fiber 1.9, Carbs 9.8, Protein 1.9

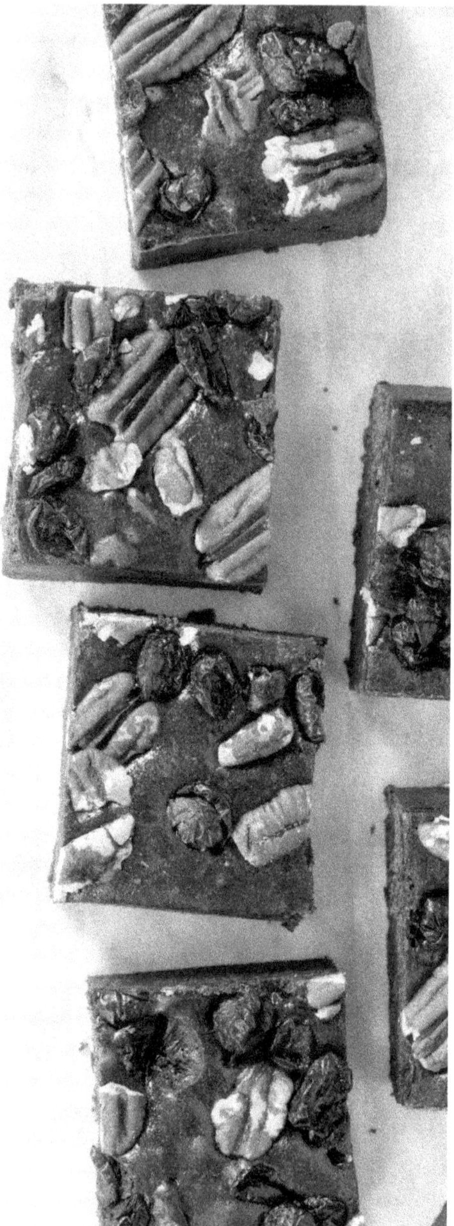

Walnut Brownies

Prep time: 20 minutes

Cook time: 25 minutes

Servings: 6

Ingredients:

- 1 egg, beaten
- ⅓ cup of cocoa powder
- 2 tablespoons erythritol
- 7 tablespoons coconut oil
- ½ teaspoon ground cinnamon
- ¼ cup coconut flour
- 2 oz walnuts, chopped
- ½ teaspoon baking powder

Method:

1. Put all ingredients in the food processor and blend until homogenous.
2. Then line the baking pan with baking paper and pour the brownie batter inside. Flatten the brownie dough and bake it at 360F for 25 minutes.
3. Then cool the cooked dessert and cut into bars.

Nutritional info per serve: Calories 237, Fat 23.3, Fiber 4.2, Carbs 12.3, Protein 4.7

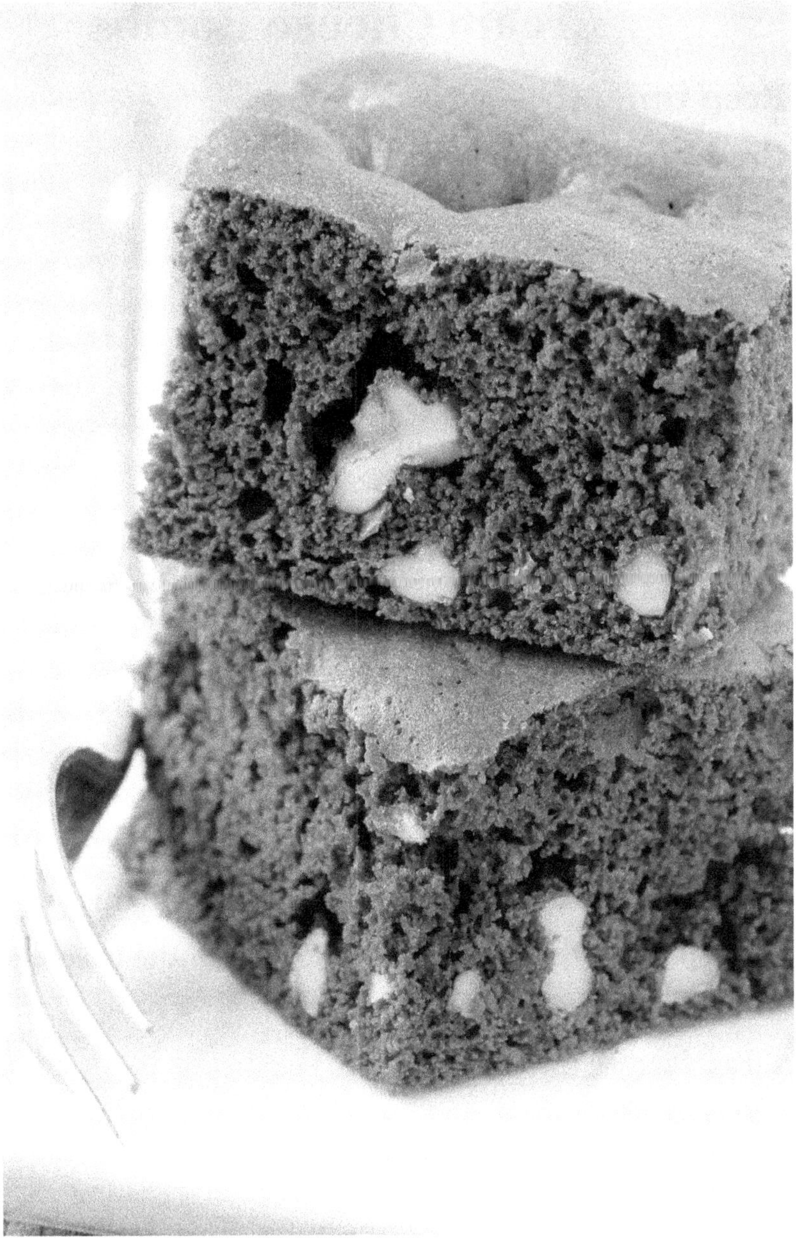

Cream Cheese Bombs

Prep time: 20 minutes

Cook time: 0 minutes

Servings:5

Ingredients:

- 5 tablespoons cream cheese
- 1 teaspoon vanilla extract
- 2 eggs, boiled, chopped
- 2 tablespoons Erythritol
- ¾ teaspoon lemon zest, grated
- 1 tablespoon coconut shred

Method:

1. Put all ingredients in the mixing bowl and mix.
2. Then make the bombs with the help of the ice cream scooper.
3. Refrigerate the cream cheese bombs for 10-15 minutes before serving.

Nutritional info per serve: Calories 73, Fat 6.2, Fiber 0.2, Carbs 7, Protein 3

Blueberries Scones

Prep time: 15 minutes

Cook time: 30 minutes

Servings: 10

Ingredients:

- ½ cup almond flour
- 1 cup blueberries
- 2 eggs, beaten
- ½ cup coconut cream
- ½ cup of coconut oil
- 5 tablespoons Erythritol
- 2 teaspoons vanilla extract
- 2 teaspoons baking powder

Method:

1. Blend all ingredients in the food processor until you get a smooth batter.
2. Pour the batter in the silicone mold and bake at 360F for 30 minutes.
3. Chill the cooked dessert well and cut into scones.

Nutritional info per serve: Calories 179, Fat 17.3, Fiber 1.2, Carbs 12.1, Protein 2.7

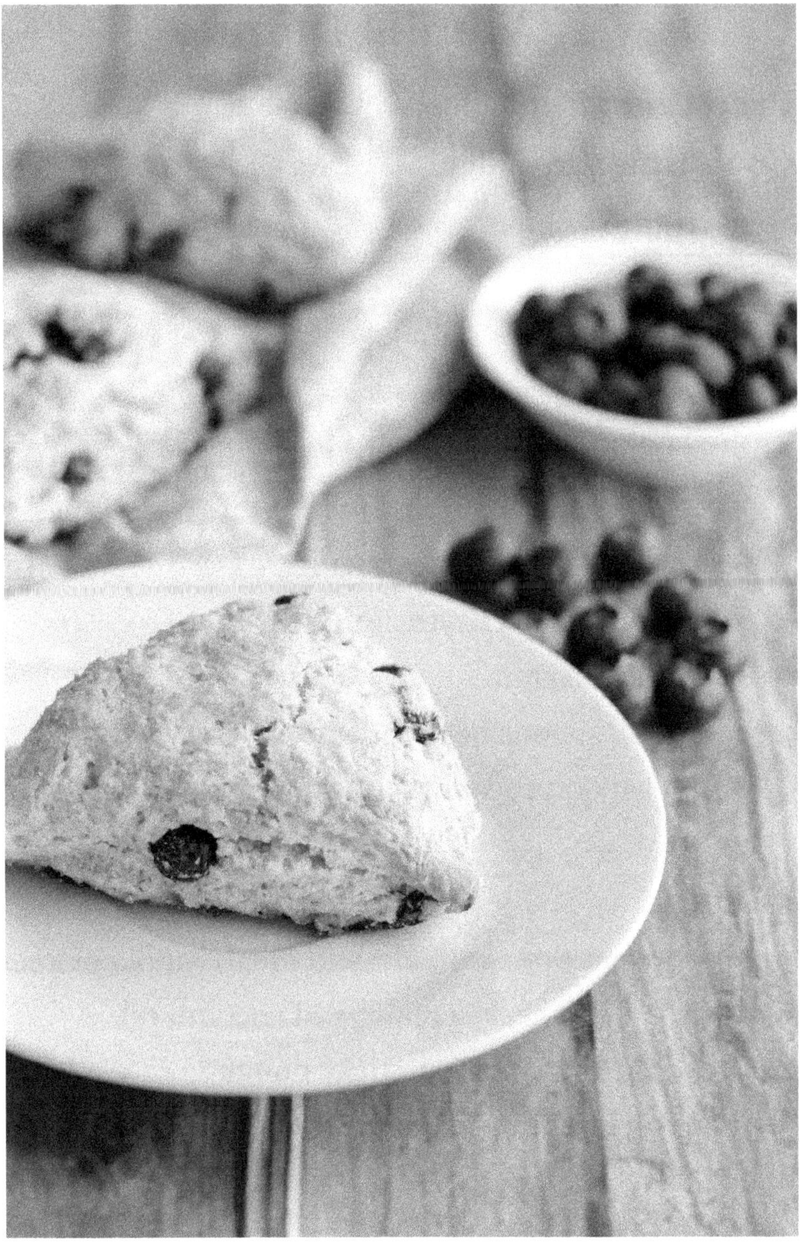

Vanilla Donuts

Prep time: 15 minutes

Cook time: 20 minutes

Servings:6

Ingredients:

- 4 tablespoons coconut flour
- 2 tablespoons almond meal
- 1 teaspoon vanilla extract
- 2 tablespoons Erythritol
- 2 eggs, beaten
- 2 tablespoons heavy cream
- 1 teaspoon coconut oil, softened

Method:

1. Mix coconut flour with almond meal, vanilla extract, Erythritol, eggs, heavy cream, and coconut oil.
2. Knead the soft and non-sticky dough.
3. Then roll it up and make the donuts with the help of the donut cutter.
4. Bake the donuts at 360F for 20 minutes.

Nutritional info per serve: Calories 98, Fat 6.4, Fiber 3.6, Carbs 11.1, Protein 3.7

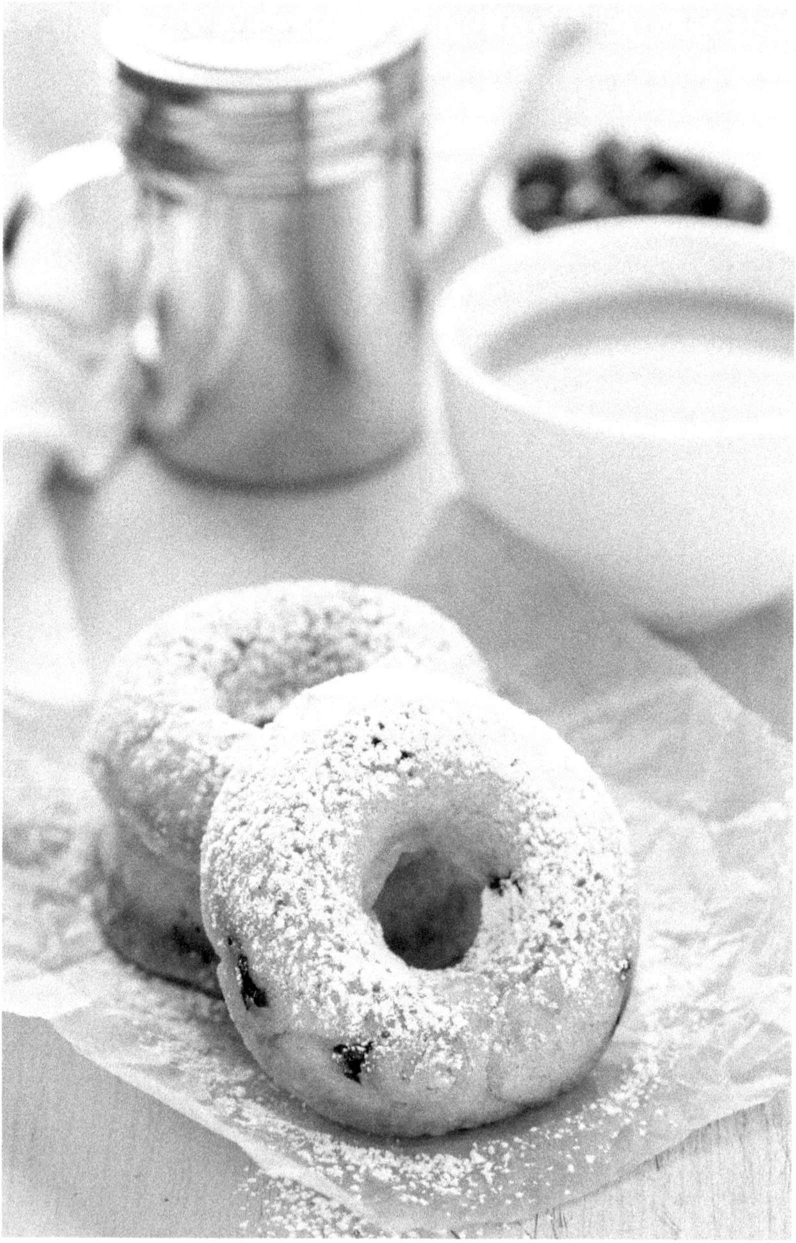

Tender Cookies

Prep time: 10 minutes

Cook time: 13 minutes

Servings: 12

Ingredients:

- 1 teaspoon vanilla extract
- ½ cup of coconut oil
- 2 eggs, beaten
- 2 tablespoons Erythritol
- 2 cups coconut flour
- 1 oz dark chocolate, chopped

Method:

1. In the mixing bowl, mix the vanilla extract with coconut oil, eggs, Erythritol, coconut flour.
2. When the mixture is homogeneous, add chopped chocolate and stir it.
3. Make the small balls from the dough and put them in the baking tray.
4. Bake the cookies at 360F for 13 minutes.

Nutritional info per serve: Calories 182, Fat 12.5, Fiber 8.1, Carbs 17.4, Protein 3.8

Keto Caramel

Prep time: 10 minutes

Cook time: 10 minutes

Servings:4

Ingredients:

- 4 teaspoons coconut oil
- ½ cup Erythritol
- ½ teaspoon vanilla extract
- 1 pecan, chopped

Method:

1. Melt the coconut oil in the saucepan.
2. Add Erythritol and vanilla extract. Melt the mixture.
3. Then remove it from the heat, add pecan, and pour the caramel in the glass jar.

Nutritional info per serve: Calories 150, Fat 16.5, Fiber 0.4, Carbs 3.6, Protein 0.4

Crustless Yogurt Cake

Prep time: 20 minutes

Cook time: 40 minutes

Servings: 12

Ingredients:

- 2 cups plain yogurt
- 2 strawberries, chopped
- 1 teaspoon vanilla extract
- 2 tablespoons gelatin
- 2 tablespoons Erythritol
- 10 tablespoons water

Method:

1. Mix water with gelatin and leave the mixture for 10 minutes.
2. Then microwave it until liquid and mix it with plain yogurt. Whisk the mixture until smooth.
3. After this, add vanilla extract, strawberries, and Erythritol.
4. Pour the yogurt mixture in the silicone mold and freeze for 30-40 minutes.

Nutritional info per serve: Calories 35, Fat 0.5, Fiber 0, Carbs 5.6, Protein 3.3

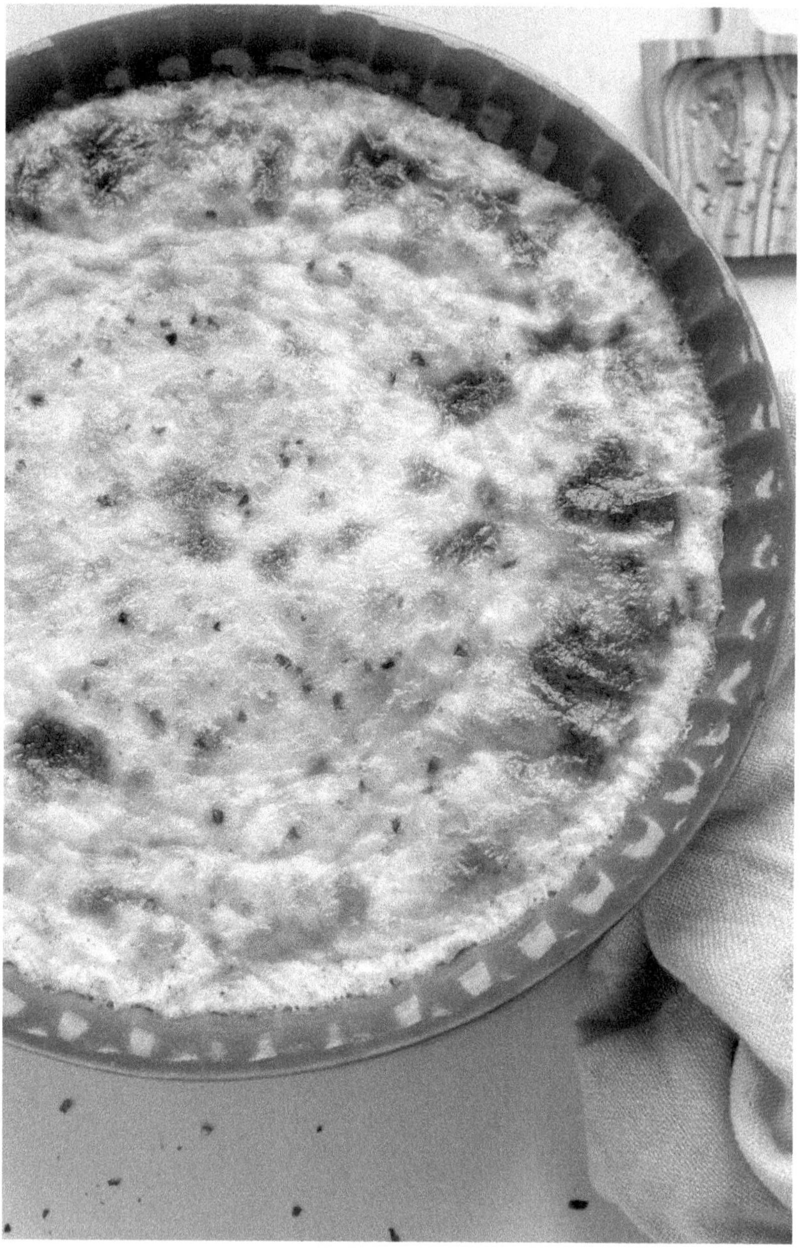

Almond Mousse

Prep time: 10 minutes

Servings:2

Ingredients:

- 4 tablespoons cream cheese
- 4 tablespoons organic almond milk
- 1 teaspoon Erythritol

Method:

1. Blend cream cheese with almond milk and Erythritol.
2. When the mixture is smooth and fluffy, transfer it in the serving glasses.

Nutritional info per serve: Calories 139, Fat 14.1, Fiber 0.7, Carbs 4.7, Protein 2.2

Cocoa Paste

Prep time: 10 minutes

Cook time: 0 minutes

Servings: 6

Ingredients:

- 2 oz butter, softened
- 4 tablespoons cocoa powder
- 1 teaspoon ground cinnamon

Method:

1. Whisk the butter with cocoa powder until fluffy and transfer in the serving bowl.
2. Top the paste with ground cinnamon.

Nutritional info per serve: Calories 7.7, Fat 8.1, Fiber 1.3, Carbs 2.3, Protein 0.8

Ricotta Bars

Prep time: 25 minutes

Cook time: 0 minutes

Servings:6

Ingredients:

- 6 tablespoons coconut oil, softened
- 6 tablespoons ricotta cheese
- 1 teaspoon vanilla extract
- 3 tablespoons Erythritol

Method:

1. Mix ricotta cheese with coconut oil.
2. When the mixture is smooth, add vanilla extract and Erythritol.
3. Stir the mixture and transfer in the baking tray. Flatten the mixture and freeze for 20 minutes.
4. Cut the cooked meal into the bars.

Nutritional info per serve: Calories 141, Fat 14.8, Fiber 0, Carbs 8.4, Protein 1.8

Stevia Pie

Prep time: 10 minutes

Cook time: 30 minutes

Servings: 4

Ingredients:

- 1 cup of coconut milk
- 1 cup almond flour
- 1 teaspoon baking powder
- 3 eggs, beaten
- 2 tablespoons liquid stevia
- 1 teaspoon vanilla extract
- Cooking spray

Method:

1. Mix coconut milk with almond flour, baking powder, eggs, liquid stevia, and vanilla extract.
2. Spray the baking pan with cooking spray from inside.
3. Pour the coconut mixture in the baking pan and bake at 350F for 30 minutes.

Nutritional info per serve: Calories 349, Fat 31.6, Fiber 4.4, Carbs 10.3, Protein 11.5

Lime Meringue

Prep time: 15 minutes

Cook time: 2.5 hours

Servings:5

Ingredients:

- 2 egg whites,
- 5 teaspoons Erythritol
- 1 teaspoon lime juice
- 1 tablespoon coconut flour

Method:

1. Whisk the egg whites until you get the soft peaks.
2. Then add Erythritol, lime juice, and coconut flour. Whisk the egg whites for 1 minute more.
3. Then line the baking tray with baking paper.
4. Make the small meringues from the egg white mixture (use the spoon) and bake them at 340F for 2.5 hours.

Nutritional info per serve: Calories 13, Fat 0.2, Fiber 0.6, Carbs 6.2, Protein 1.7

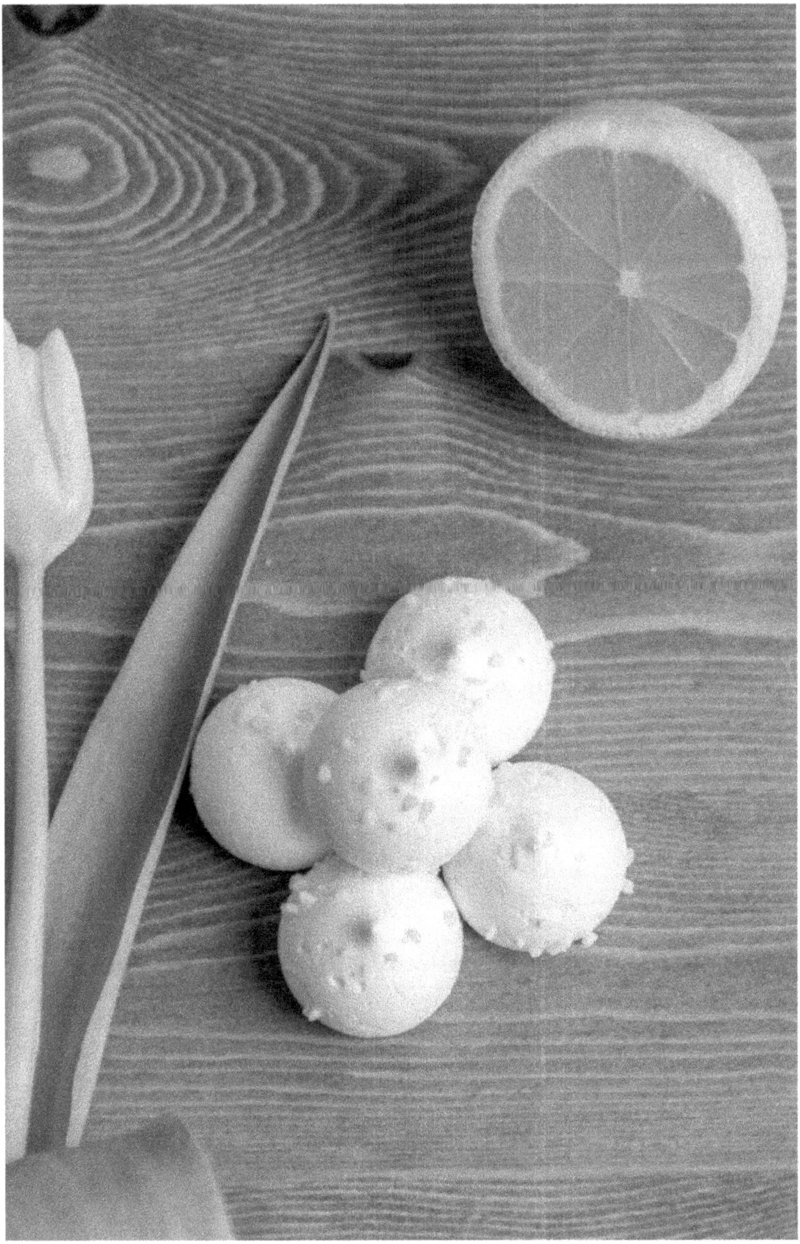

Cinnamon Buns

Prep time: 20 minutes

Cook time: 25 minutes

Servings: 8

Ingredients:

- ½ cup coconut flour
- ½ cup almond meal
- 1 teaspoon baking powder
- 1 tablespoon Erythritol
- 1 tablespoon ground cinnamon
- 2 tablespoons butter, softened
- ¼ cup of coconut milk

Method:

1. In the mixing bowl, mix coconut flour with almond meal, baking powder, Erythritol, and knead the dough.
2. Then roll it up and spread with softened butter.
3. After this, sprinkle the dough with ground cinnamon and roll it.
4. Cut the roll into buns and put in the non-stick baking pan in one layer.

5. Bake the dessert at 355F for 25 minutes or until the buns are light brown.

Nutritional info per serve: Calories 110, Fat 8.4, Fiber 4.4, Carbs 9.6, Protein 2.5

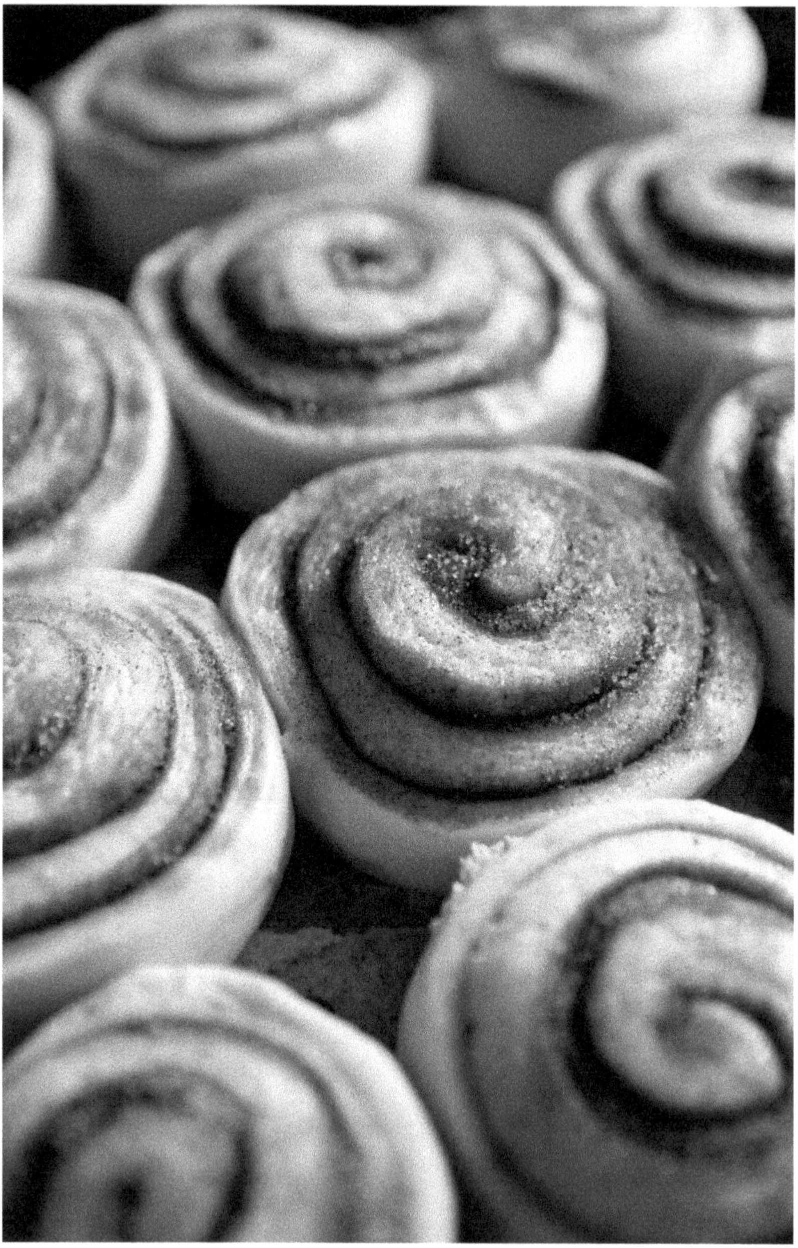

Coconut Pie

Prep time: 10 minutes

Cook time: 30 minutes

Servings:10

Ingredients:

- ½ cup coconut flour
- 1 tablespoon butter
- 1 egg, beaten
- ¾ teaspoon salt
- ½ cup ricotta cheese
- ½ cup coconut cream
- 4 tablespoons Erythritol
- 1 teaspoon vanilla extract
- 1 tablespoon coconut oil

Method:

1. Put all ingredients in the mixing bowl and stir until smooth.
2. Then transfer the prepared batter in the non-stick baking pan and flatten it if needed.
3. Bake the pie at 360F for 30 minutes.

4. Then chill the cooked dessert well and cut into servings.

Nutritional info per serve: Calories 98, Fat 7.4, Fiber 2.7, Carbs 11.4, Protein 3

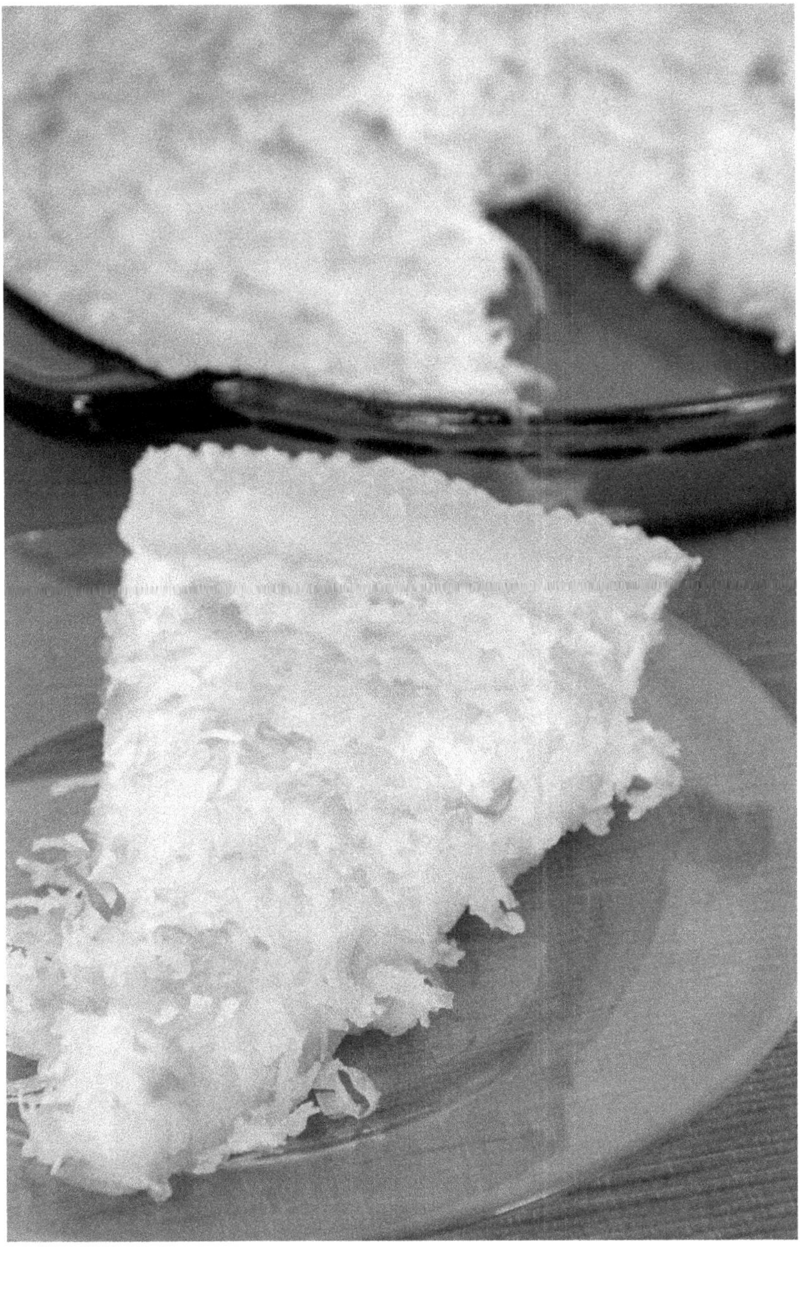

Coconut Custard

Prep time: 10 minutes

Cook time: 15 minutes

Servings: 8

Ingredients:

- 1⅓ cup of coconut milk
- 4 tablespoons lime zest
- 6 eggs, beaten
- 5 tablespoons Erythritol
- 1 teaspoon lime juice

Method:

1. Mix coconut milk with lime zest, eggs, and Erythritol.
2. Bring the mixture to boil. Stir it constantly.
3. Then pour the custard in the serving glasses and cool to the room temperature.
4. Sprinkle the dessert with lime juice.

Nutritional info per serve: Calories 302, Fat 29.5, Fiber 2.8, Carbs 16.3, Protein 6.7

Almond Bun

Prep time: 15 minutes

Cook time: 35 minutes

Servings:6

Ingredients:

- 3 tablespoons coconut oil
- 1 cup almond flour
- 1 oz almonds, chopped
- ½ teaspoon baking powder
- ½ teaspoon apple cider vinegar
- 1 tablespoon Erythritol
- 2 tablespoons almond meal
- 1 tablespoon ricotta cheese

Method:

1. In the mixing bowl, mix coconut oil with almond flour, baking powder, apple cider vinegar, and almond meal. Knead the dough.
2. Then roll up the dough.
3. In the separated bowl, mix ricotta cheese, Erythritol, and almonds.

4. Spread the ricotta mixture over the dough. Roll the dough into roll.
5. Cut the roll into 6 buns and bake at 360F for 35 minutes.

Nutritional info per serve: Calories 202, Fat 18.2, Fiber 2.6, Carbs 7.8, Protein 5.3

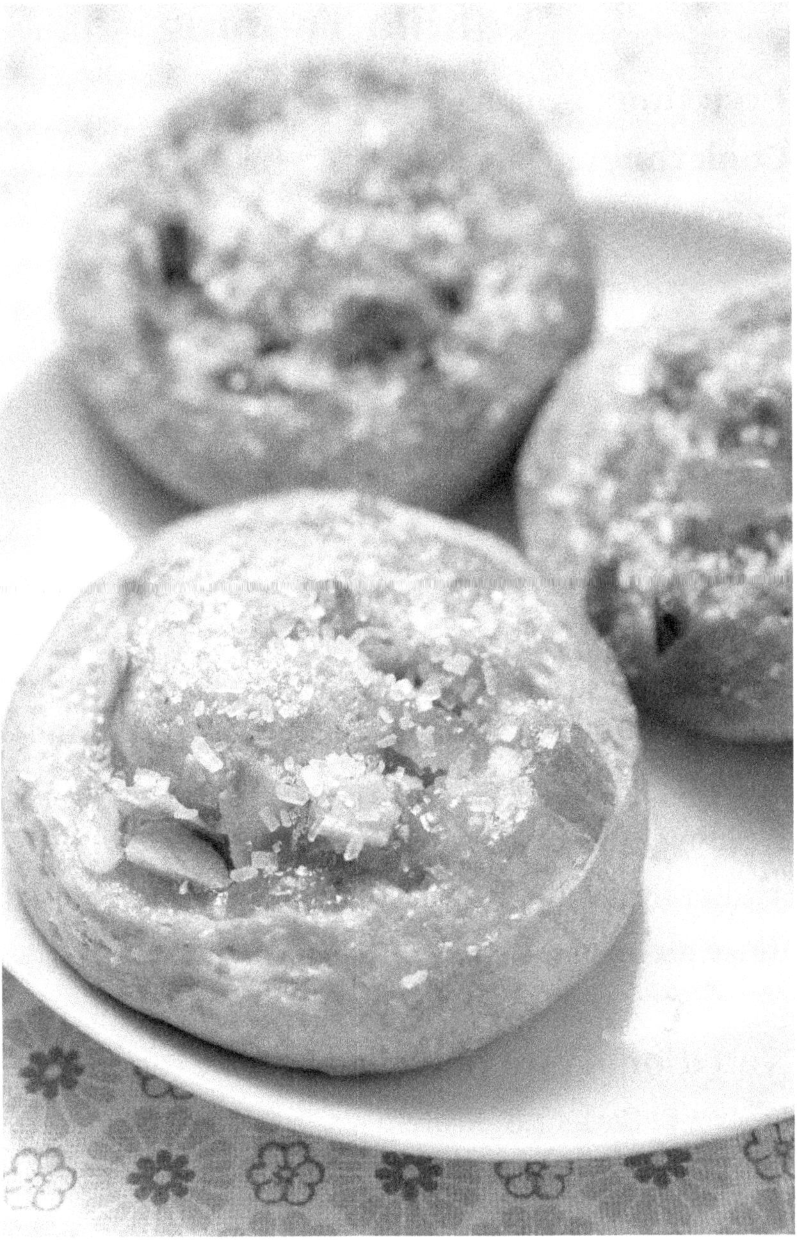

Vanilla Topping

Prep time: 15 minute

Cook time: 10 minutes

Servings: 6

Ingredients:

- ½ cup heavy cream
- 2 tablespoons Erythritol
- 1 teaspoon vanilla extract

Method:

1. Being the heavy cream to boil. Add Erythritol and vanilla extract.
2. Simmer the mixture for 5 minutes.
3. After this, chill the cooked topping and store it in the fridge for up to 4 days.

Nutritional info per serve: Calories 202, Fat 18.2, Fiber 2.6, Carbs 7.8, Protein 5.3

Notes

Lightning Source UK Ltd.
Milton Keynes UK
UKHW020657040822
406842UK00009B/628